Teeth Shouldn't Hurt

Dental Consultant: Michael Zuk DDS

Original Cartoon & Story: Yar   Guest Cartoonist: Steven Pileggi

Introduction for Parents

The 'Toothache Guy' finally decided to accept a role in a children's book about his favorite topic. In this book he is playing a character named Tommy in honor of a couple dudes with the same name. One is Tom Watson (not to be confused with the golf pro), the famous author of 'Man Shoes' and friend of the original cartoonist. The other Tom is Dr. Tom Orent, who was the first to recognize the power of Yar's little cartoon character and introduced him to thousands of dentists.

The basic idea is children need to know that teeth need to be cared for over a lifetime to avoid toothaches, to eat properly and to look their best. They also need to become friendly with their dental professionals and have problems treated early before they develop complications. Contrary to what some believe, the first set of teeth are important. Regular dental care before it hurts whenever possible is always the best way to introduce your child to the dentist. Some dentist rules that some parents do not understand include the need for parents to remain out of sight of the child being treated. You may be asked to wait in the reception room because cooperation levels are usually better that way.

Sedation is sometimes helpful and special instructions will be provided. Avoid the use of words that have negative connotations related to upcoming treatment and simply say the dentist is going to fix the problem. Never use the threat of a dental appointment as a form of punishment or you can create a phobia that can last a lifetime. If you & your family are overdue for a dental check-up and cleaning, find a good dentist and make it part of a healthy routine. To learn more helpful hints about dental care and some fun updates from the Toothache Guy visit www.TeethShouldntHurt.com.

PS. This is an activity book so it's OK to use crayons and pencils to mark it up.

How else can we inspire more cartoonists?

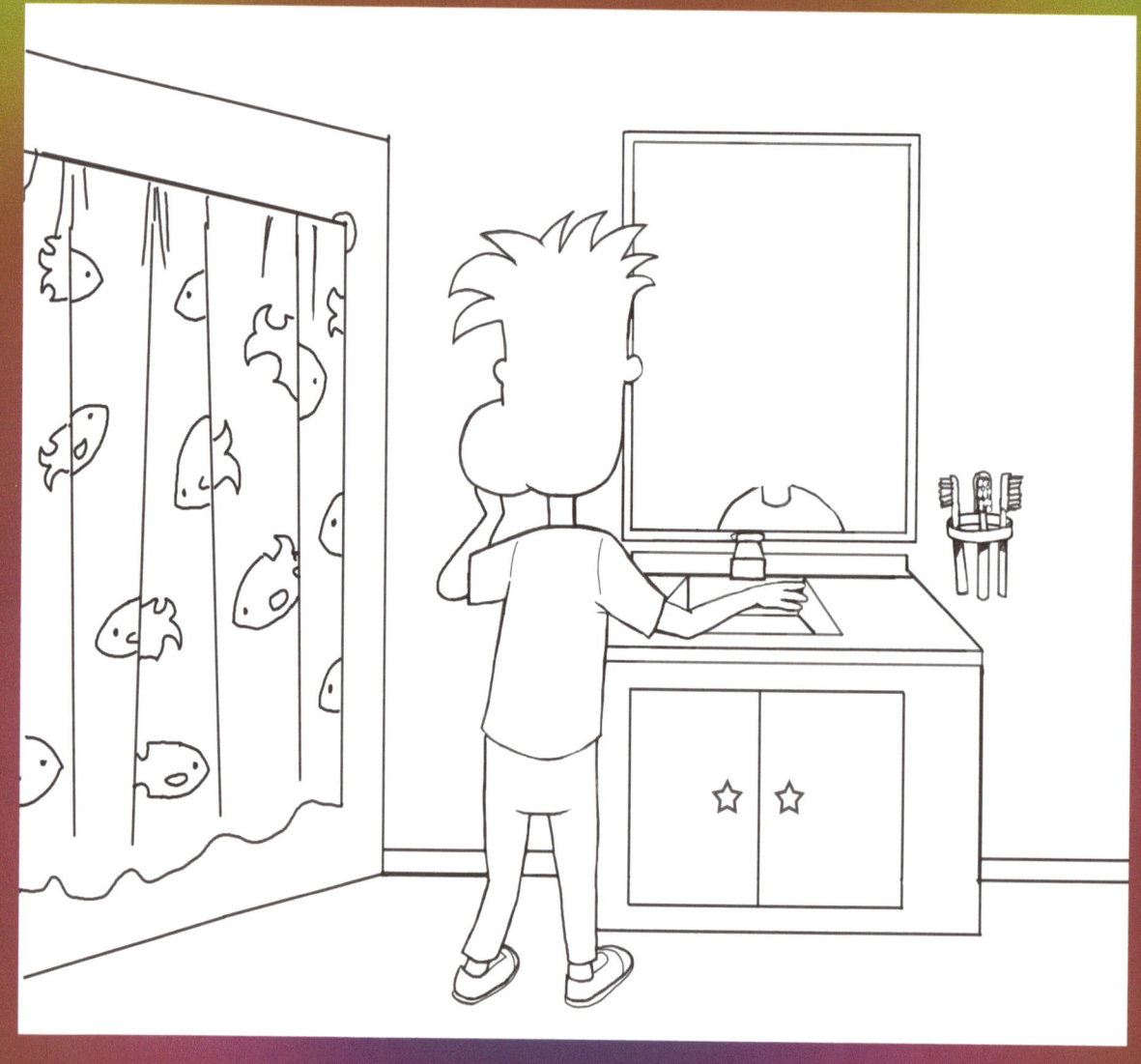

Can you draw Tommy's face in the mirror?

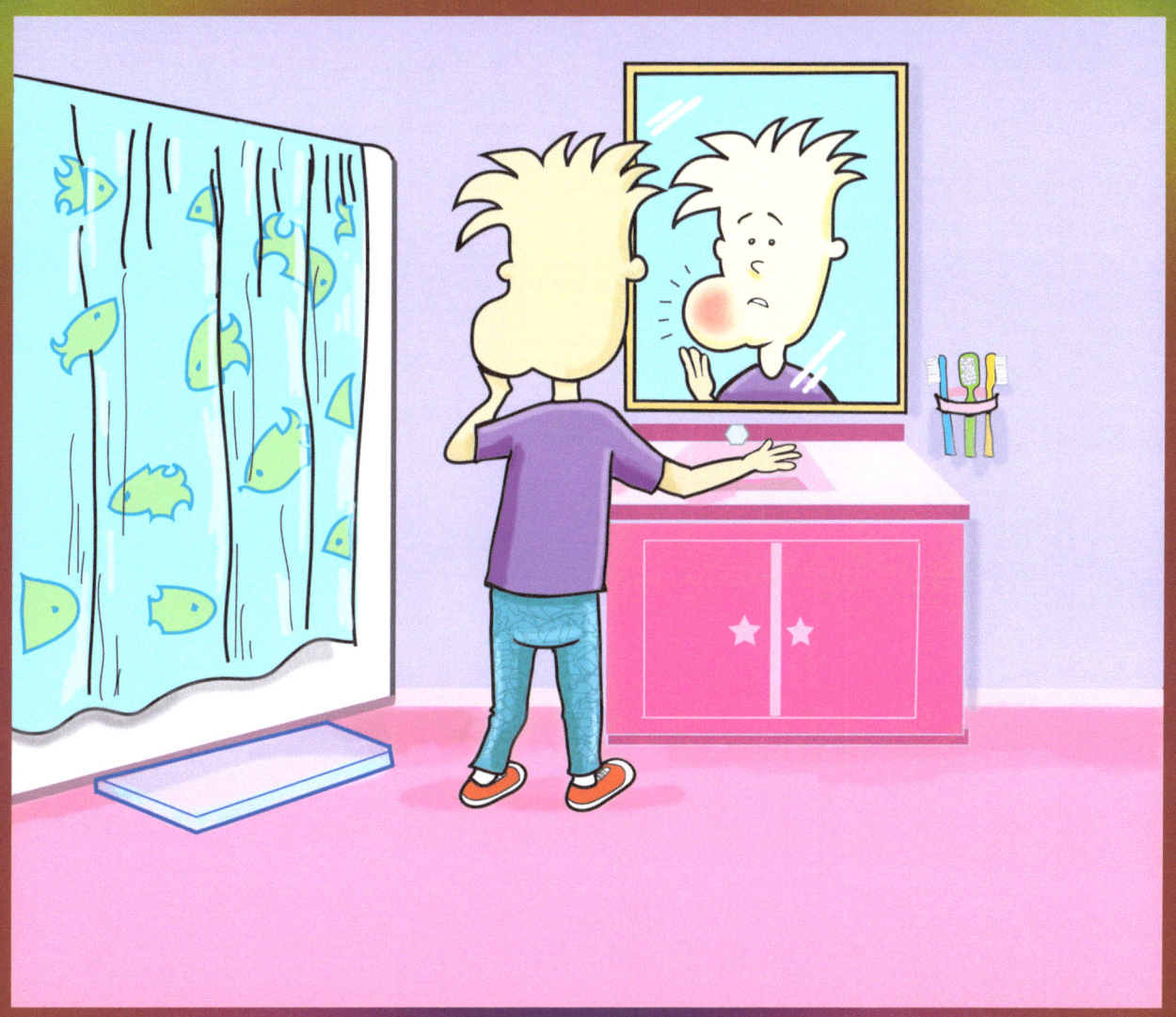

One morning Tommy woke up with a swelling on his face. It felt huge...it was warm, tender and it hurt to touch. A few weeks ago he had a toothache. Tommy had a tooth that was sensitive to sweets and hot and cold drinks. Then the tooth started to hurt a little when he chewed on it.
Tommy should have told his parents about it.

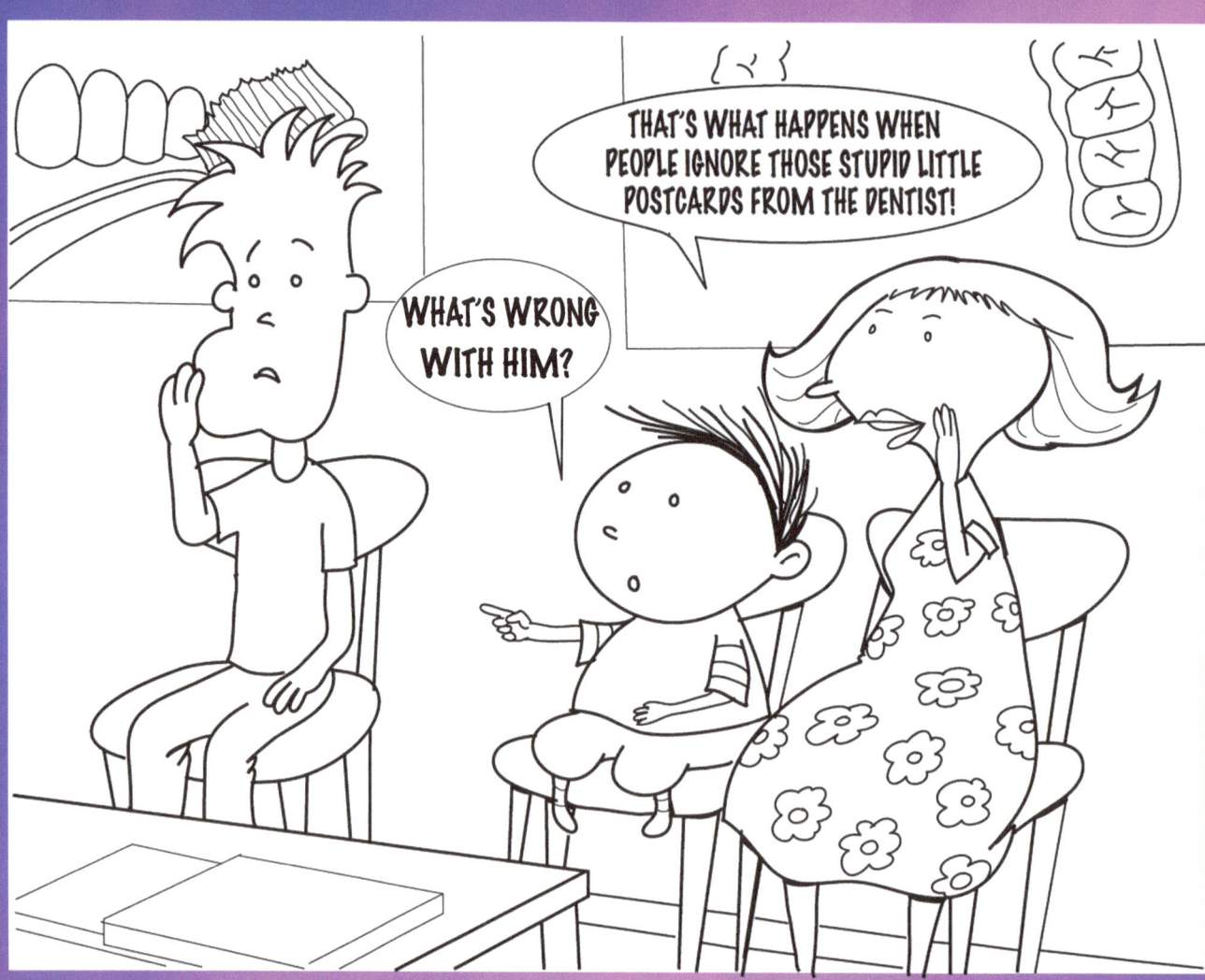

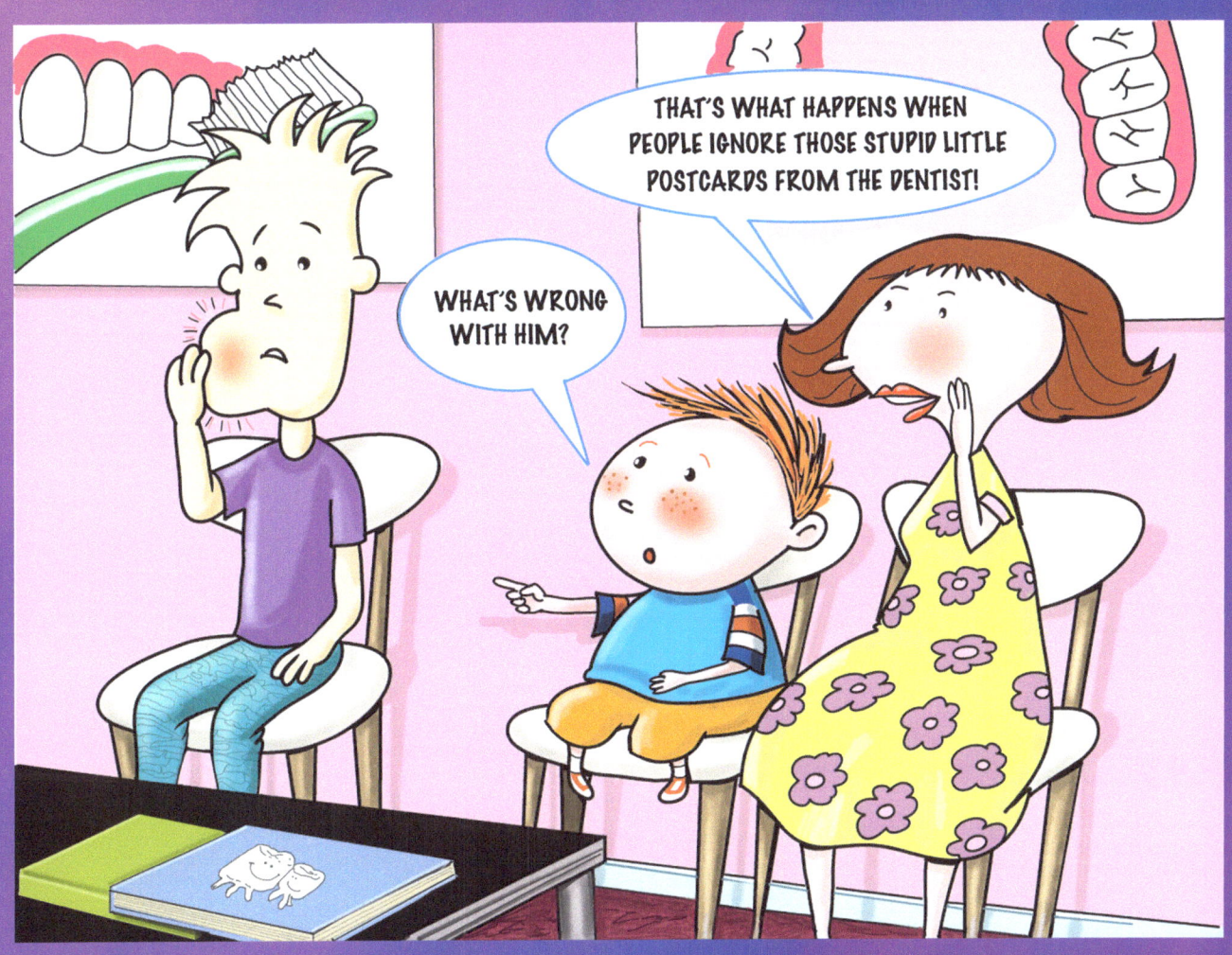

His mom called the dentist's office and they said they would fit him in right away. While in the waiting room another kid noticed Tommy's swollen face and asked his mother what the lump could be. They whispered and Tommy couldn't hear what they were saying.

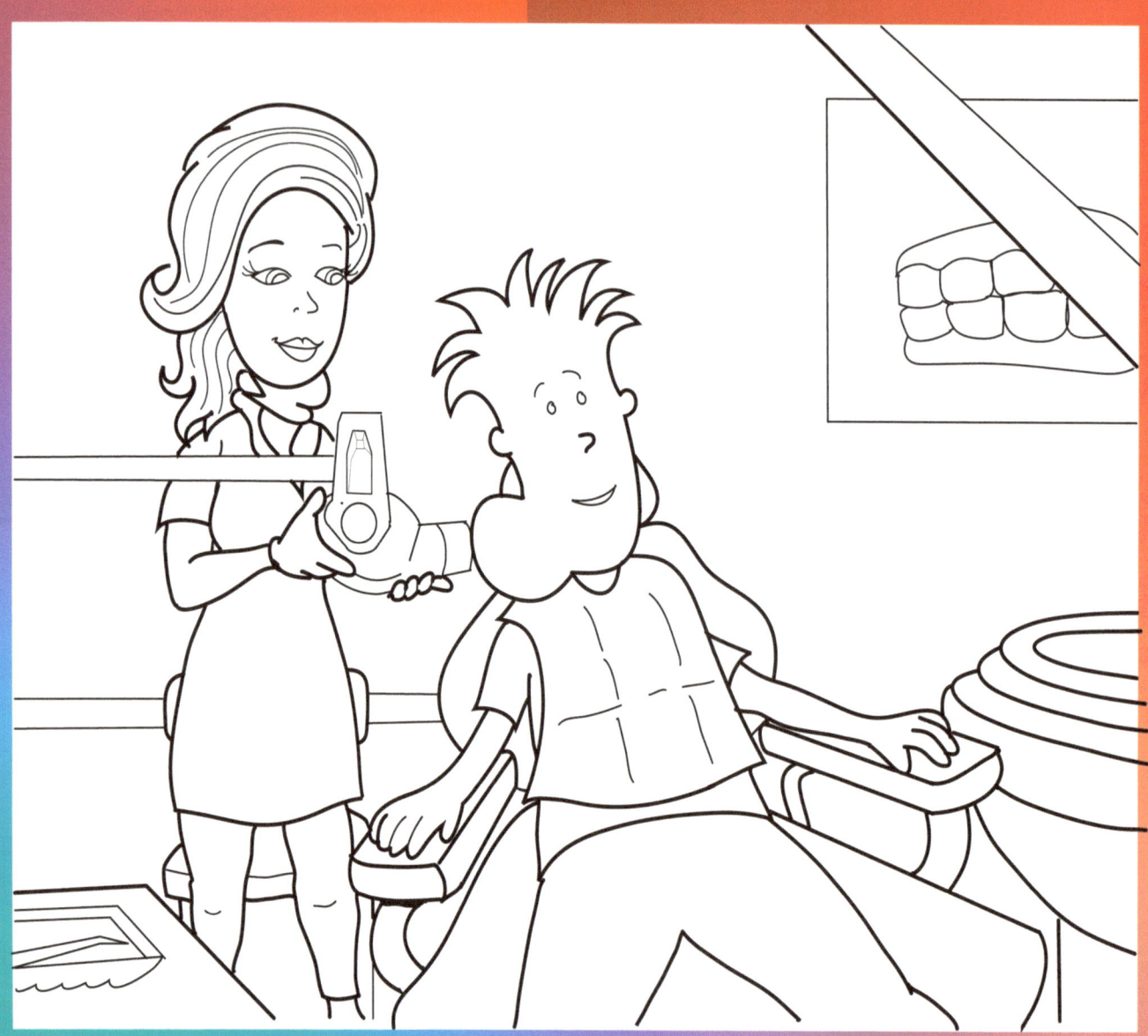

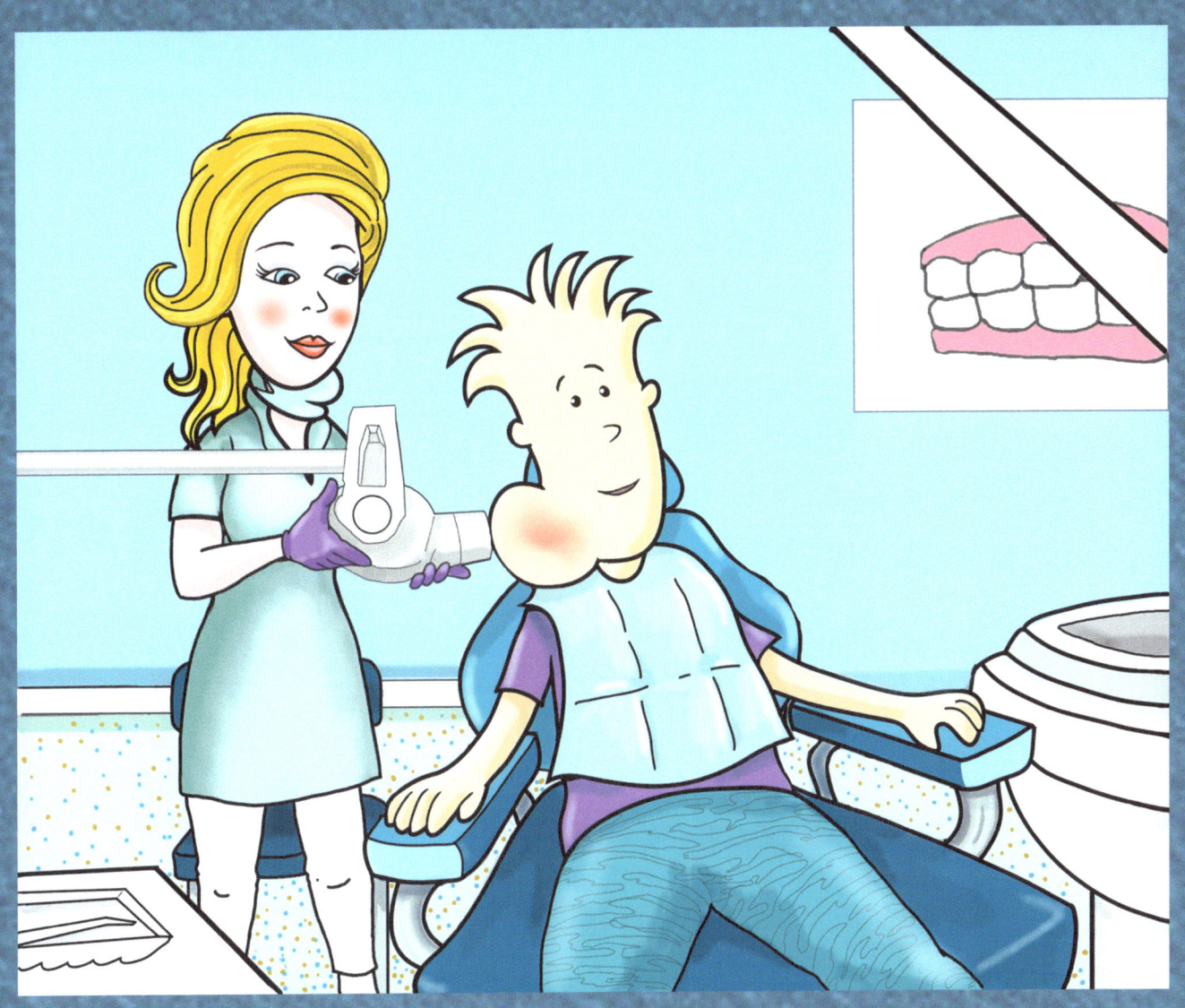

The dental assistant called Tommy's name and brought
him back to the room with a big dental chair. She took
an X-ray picture of the tooth that was hurting.

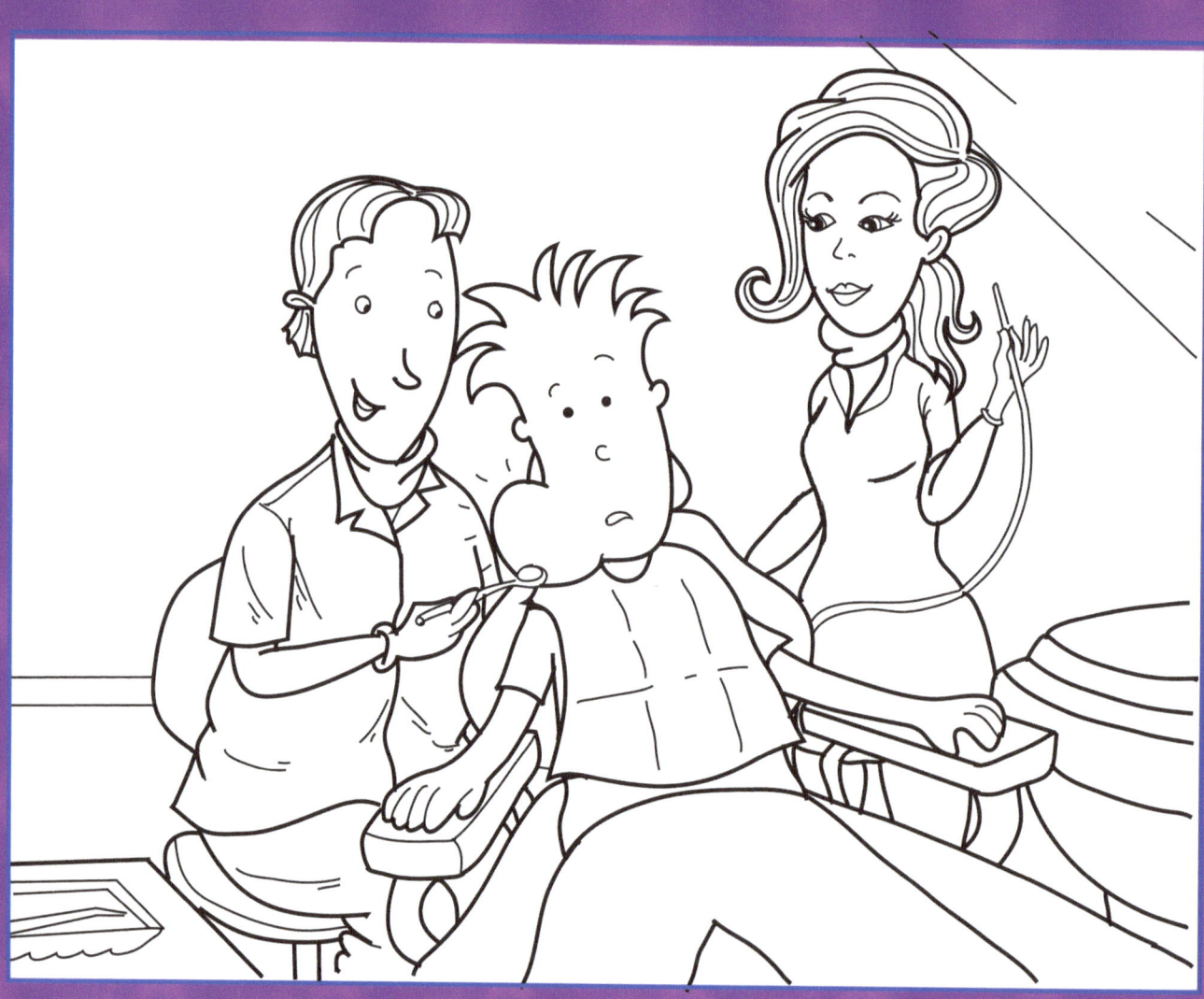

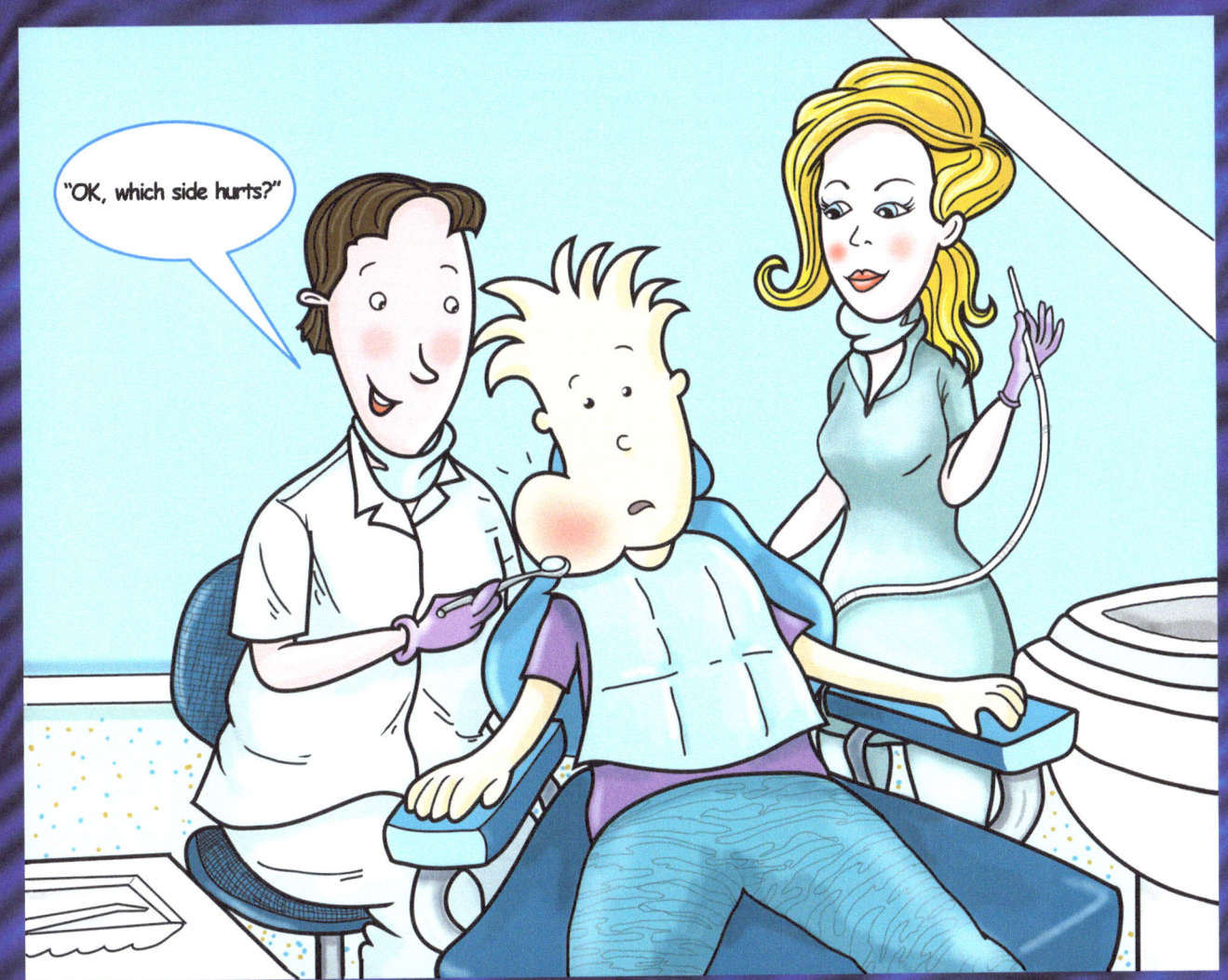

The dentist promised to do his best to fix the problem so it wouldn't bother him anymore.

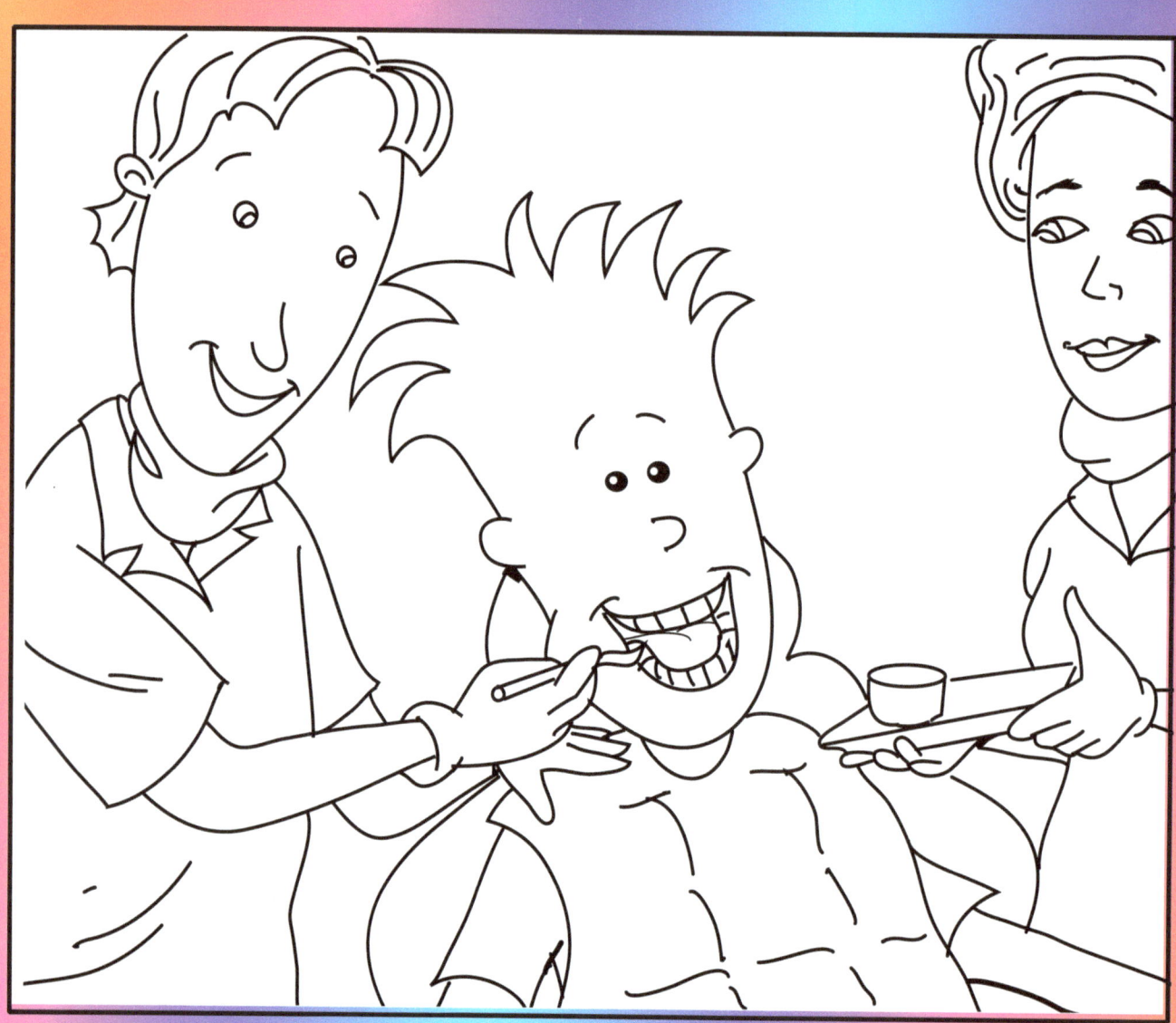

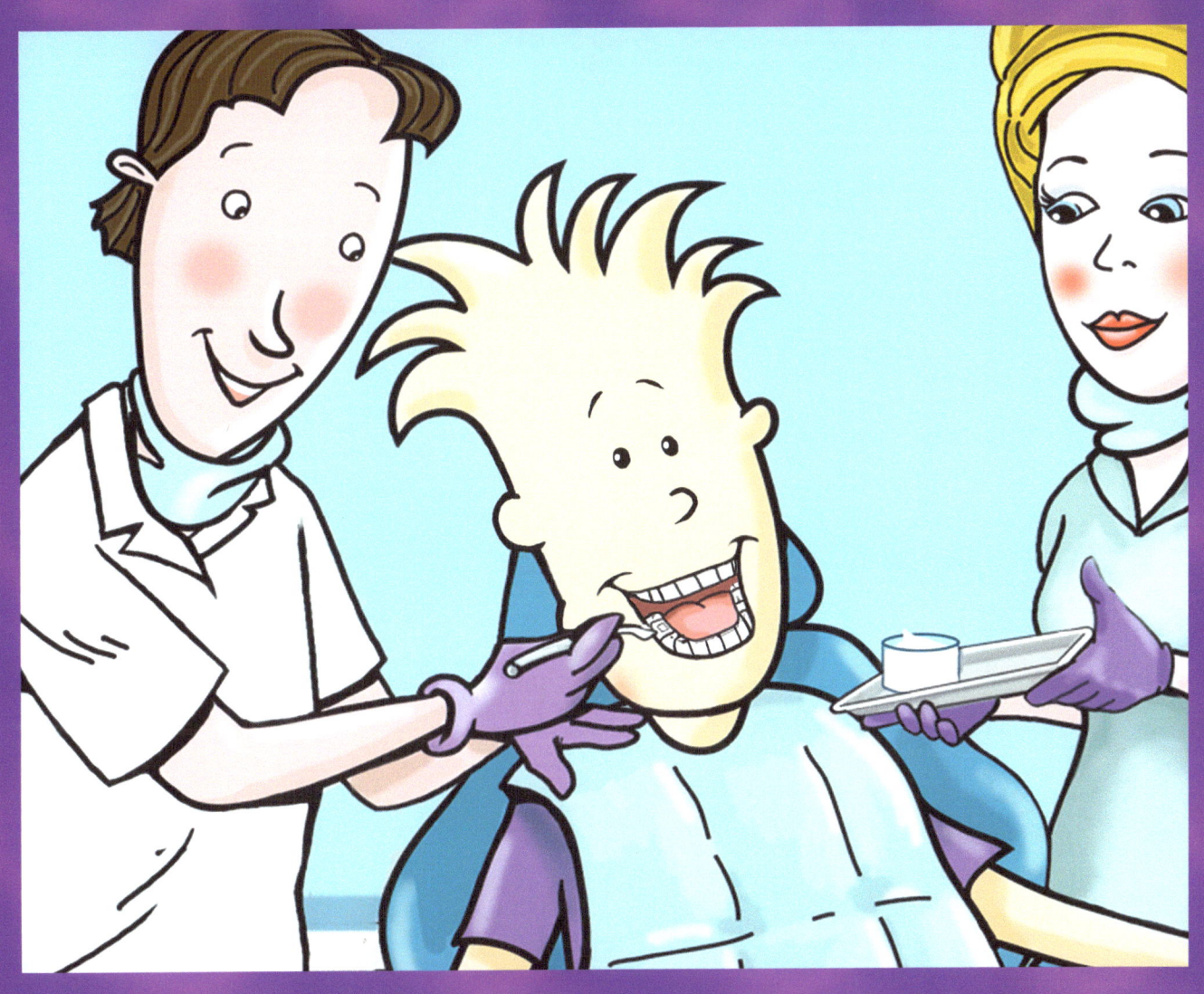

Tommy was surprised how fast the dentist was able to fix his tooth. His mouth felt fuzzy and weird, and the dental assistant warned him to be careful to avoid biting his lip while his mouth was sleeping from the freezing.

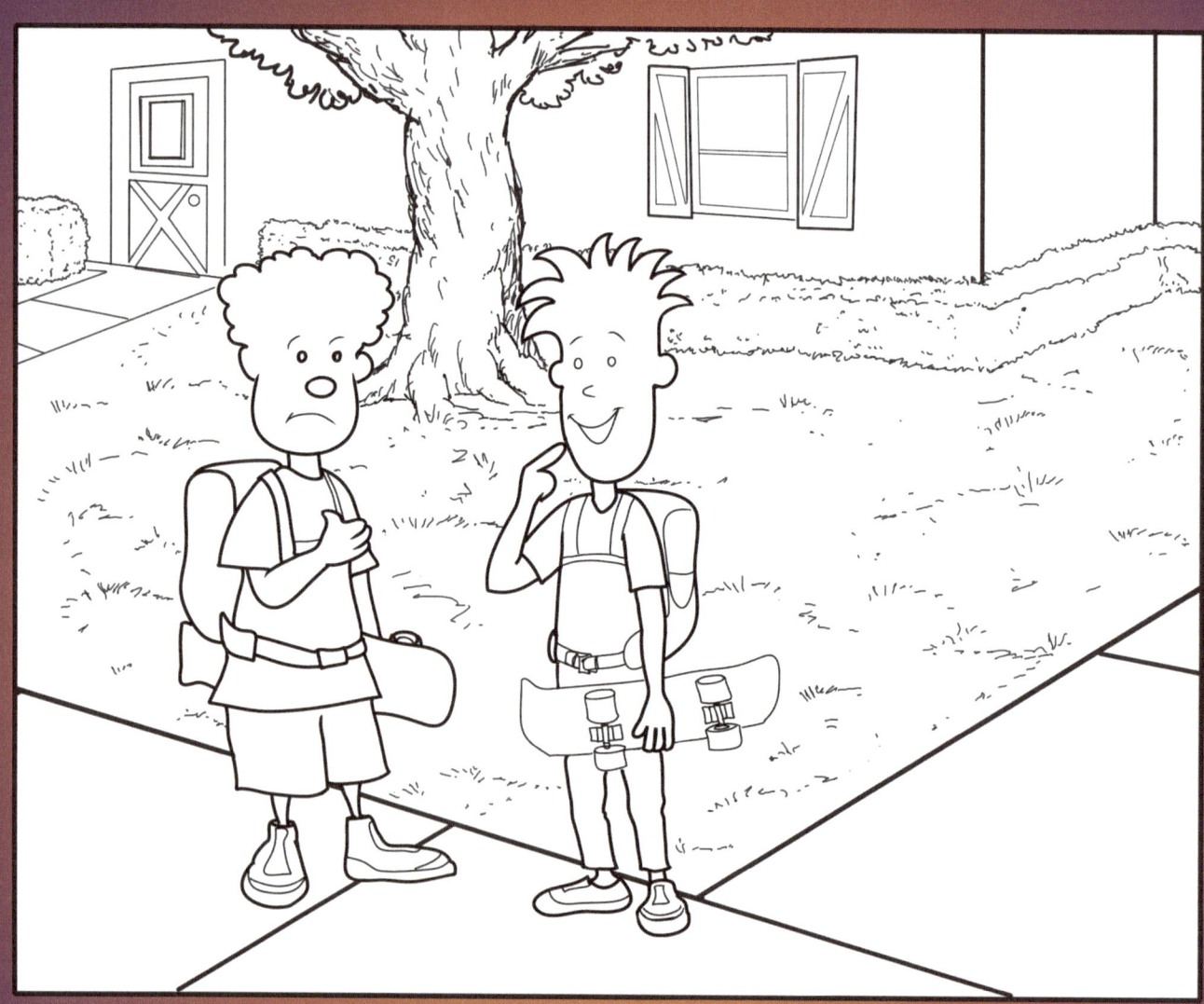

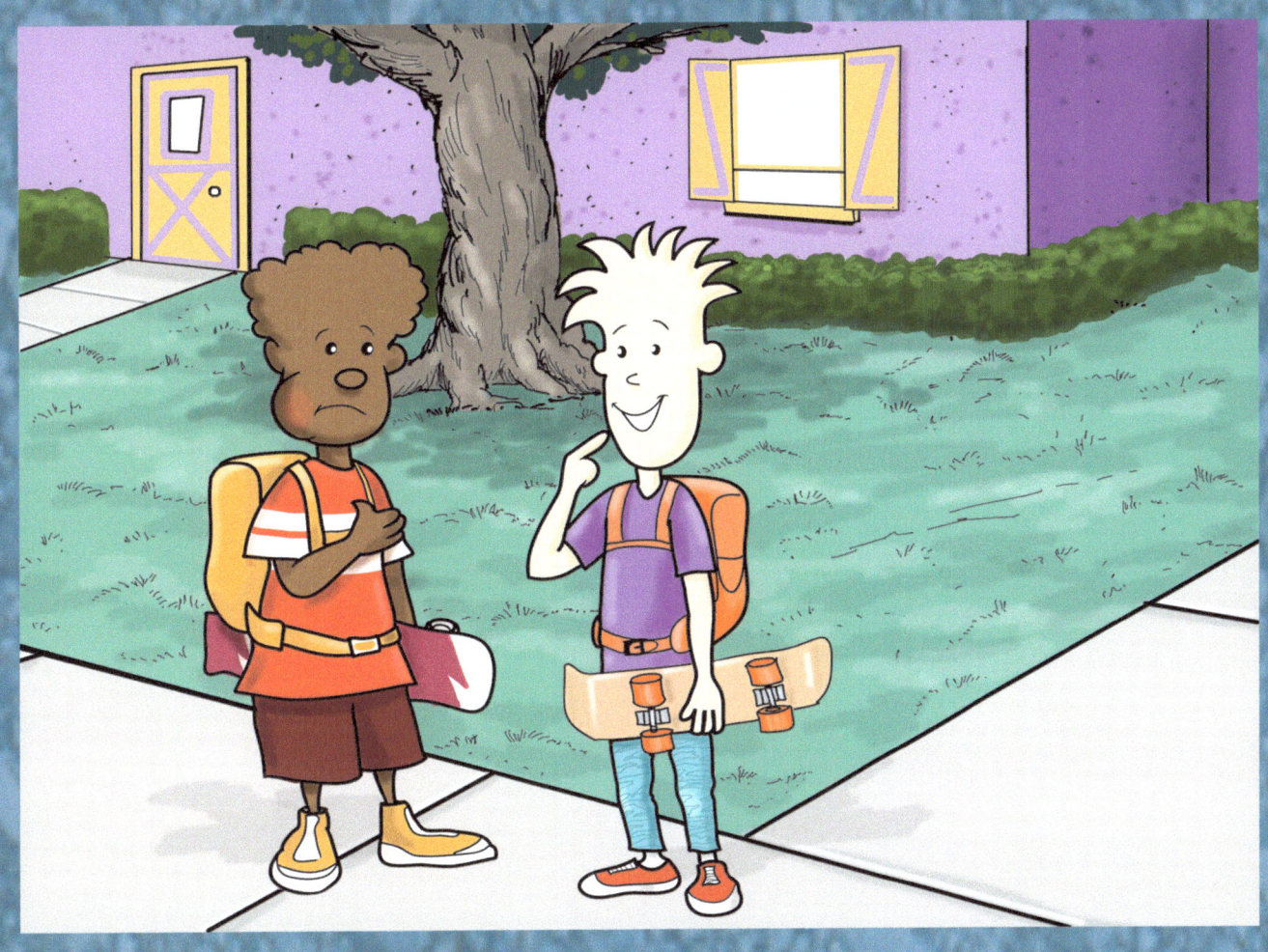

A few days later Tommy's swelling was almost gone. After school he met up with a buddy. His friend Brad looked like he had the exact same problem and Tommy told him the story of how the dentist was able to help. He told Brad to have his mom call the dental office to try to get in for an appointment before it got worse.

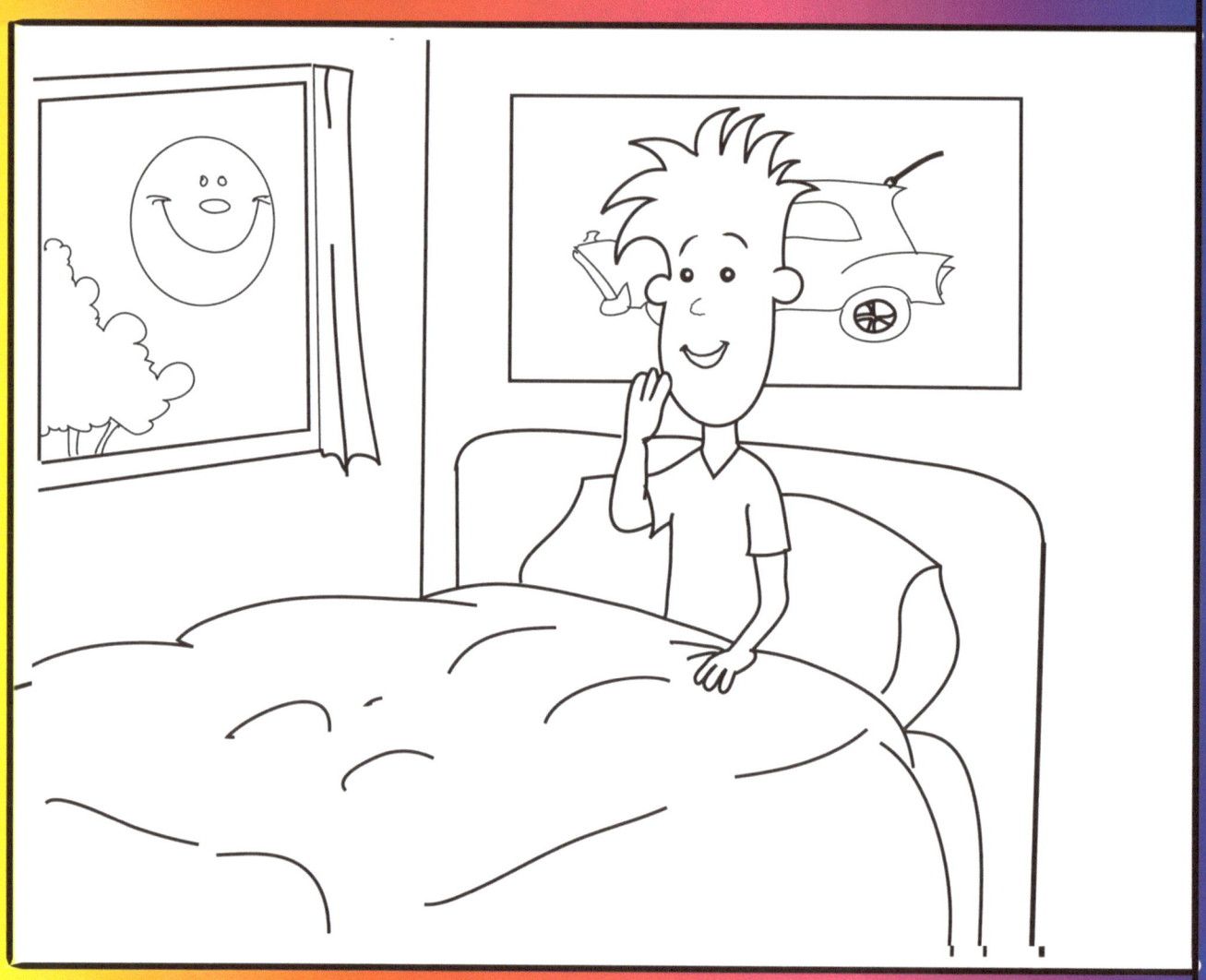

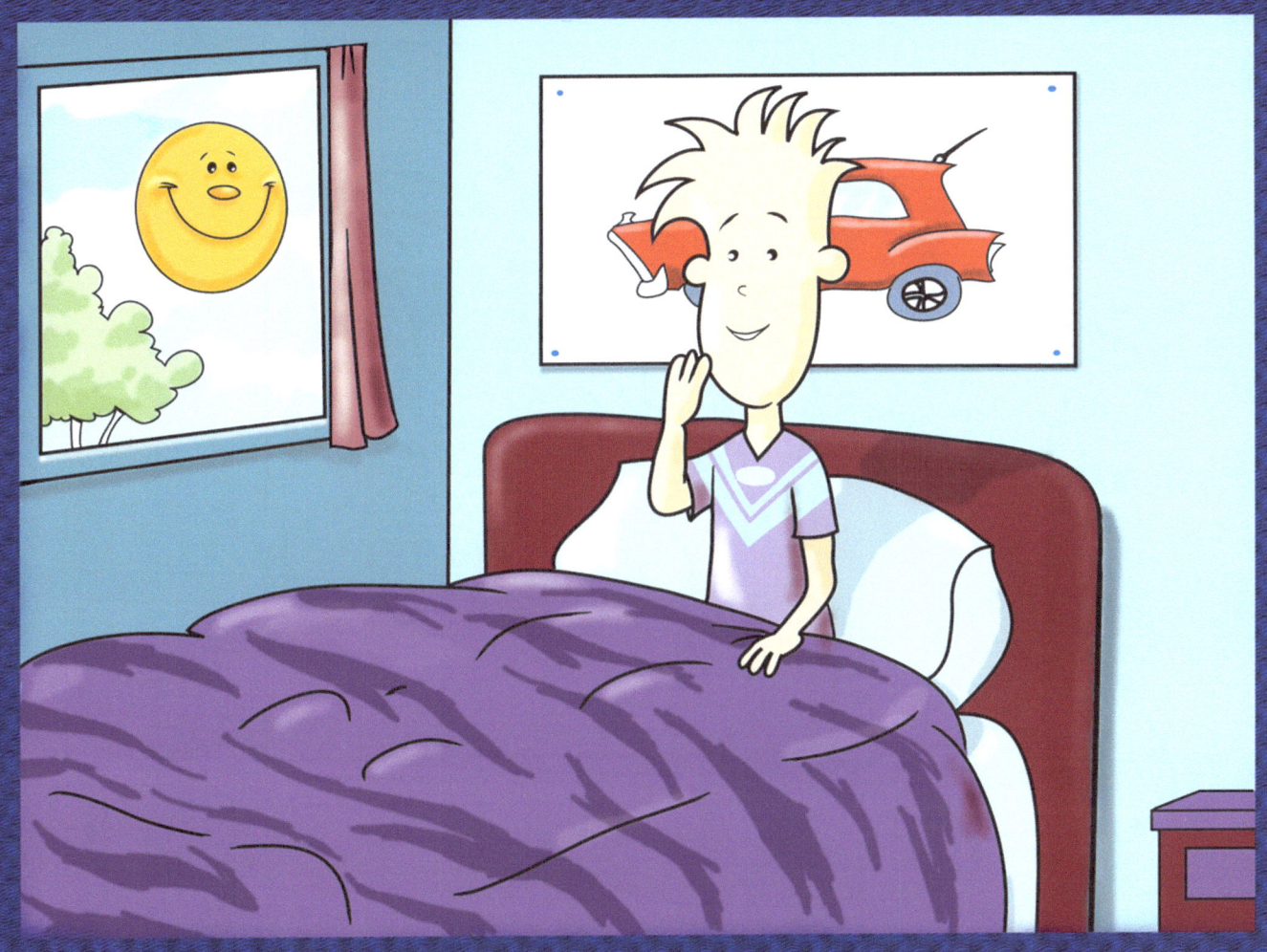

Tommy woke up and felt fine, but something was odd.
A new tooth had grown in beside the others and it
didn't fit in his mouth.

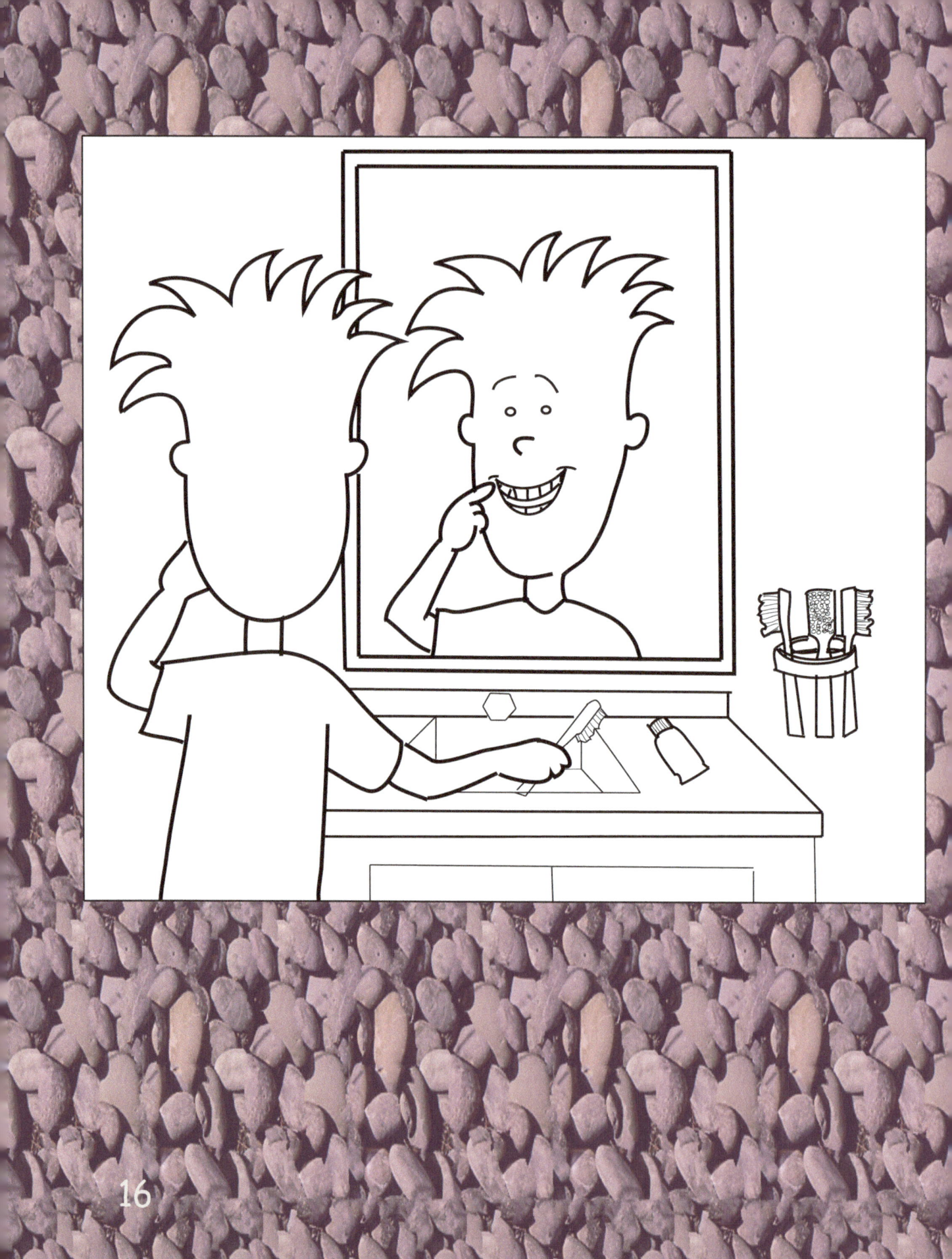

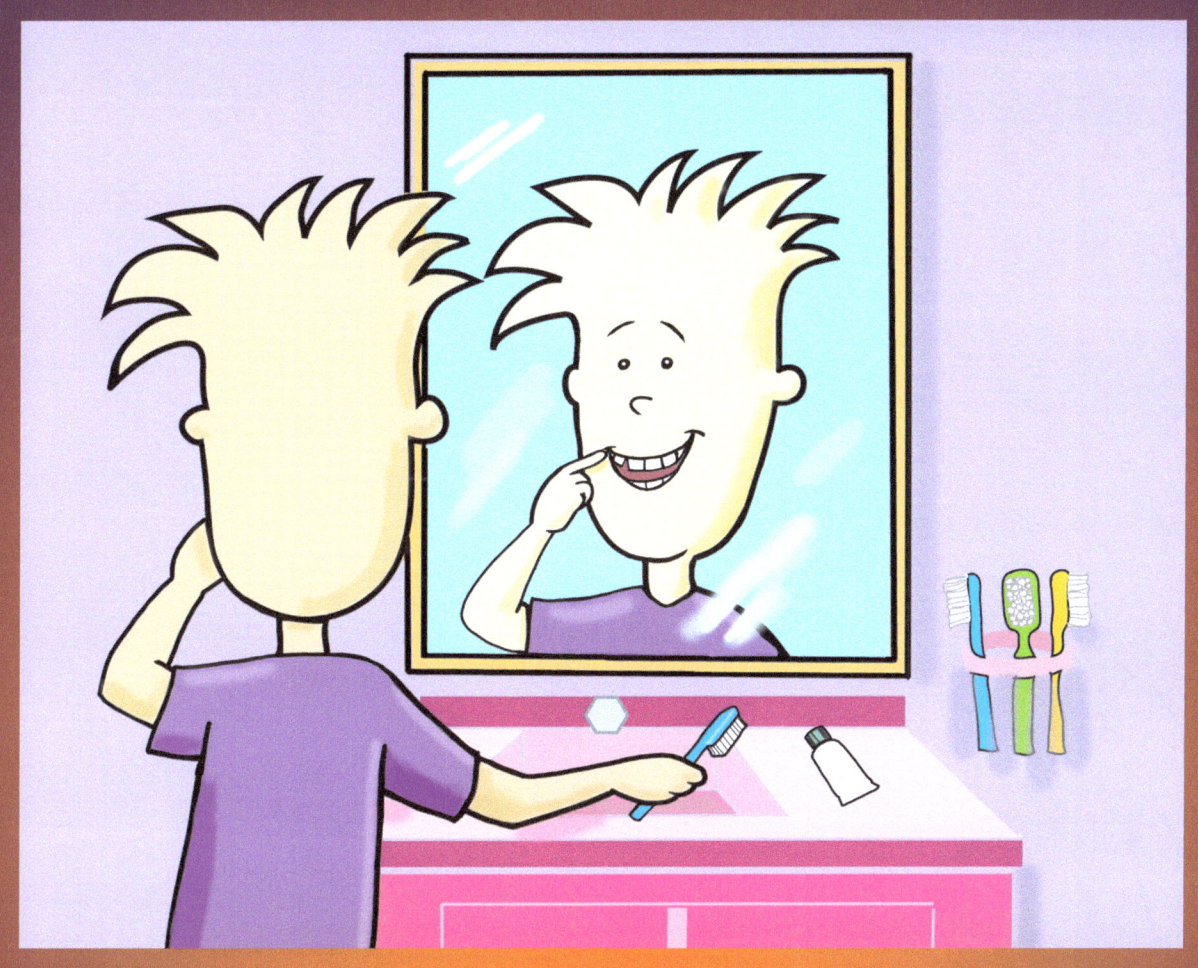

The new tooth was a little crooked but Tommy wasn't worried. He brushed and flossed his teeth, and was careful to take more time than he used to.

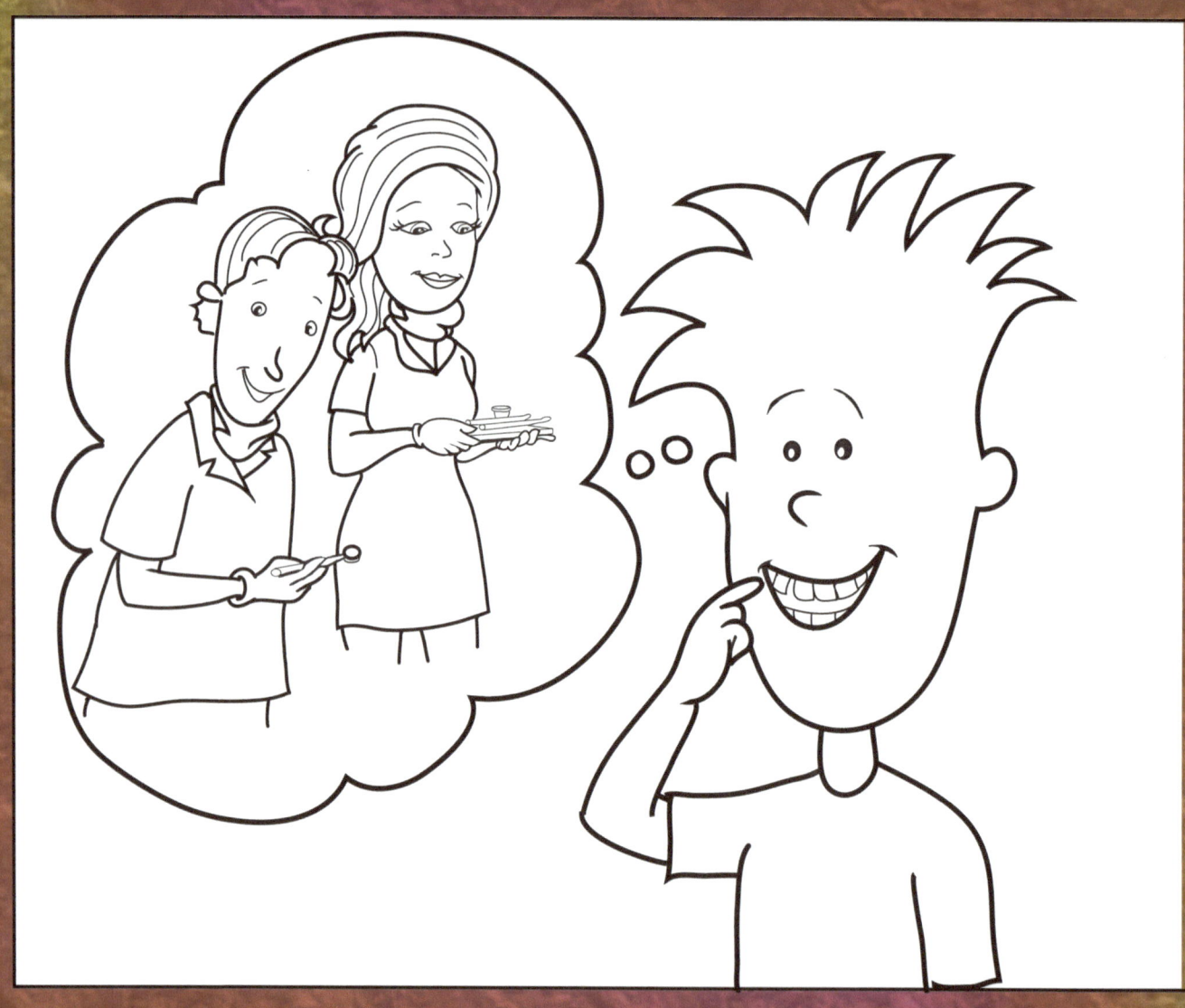

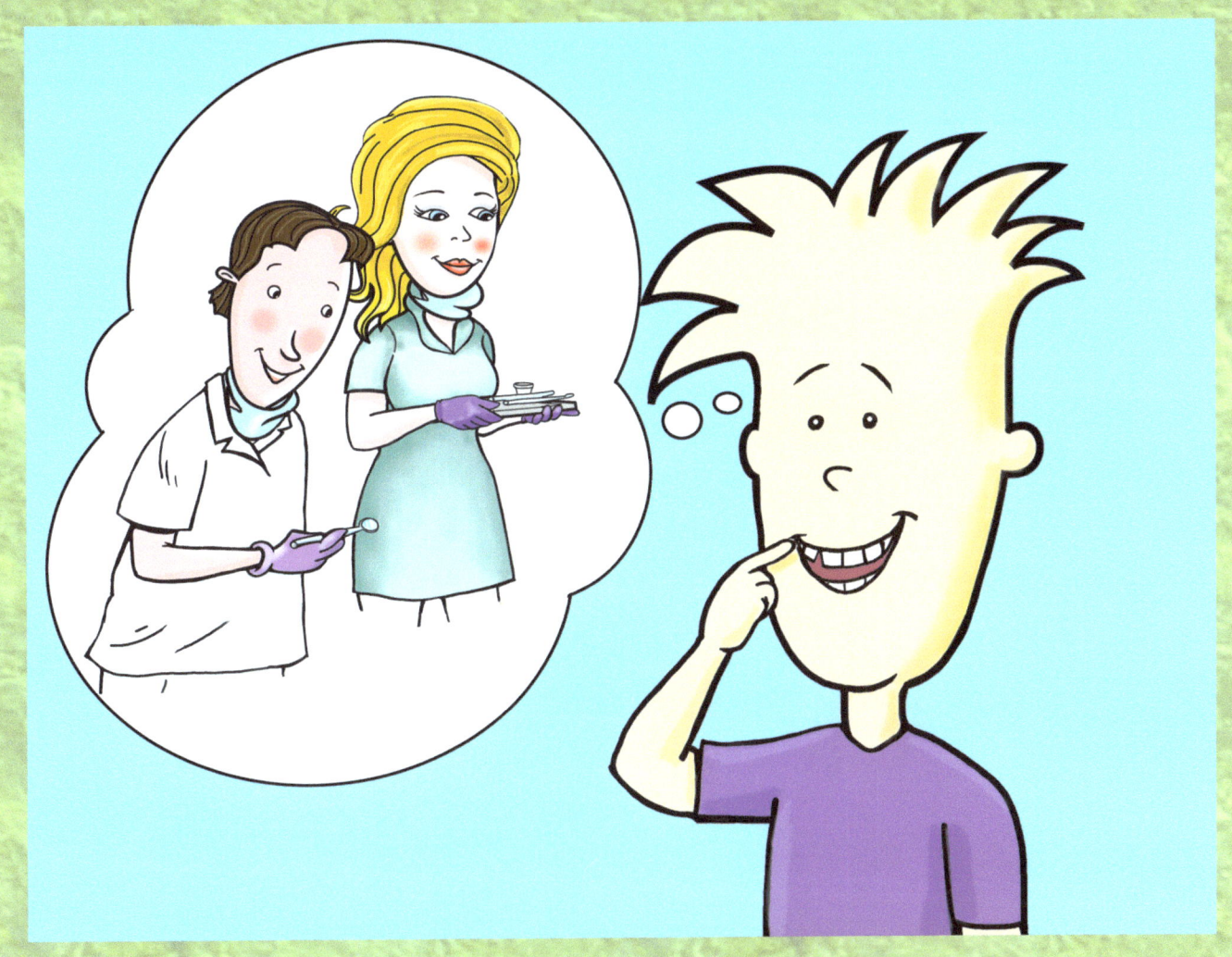

Tommy thought he should tell his parents about his new tooth. He was happy that he could visit the office and maybe even get another prize for being a good helper.

Fun Facts about Teeth

Teeth are composed of an outer shell of
a hard material called enamel.

Primary teeth are sometimes called baby teeth,
deciduous teeth or milk teeth.

Most people have 20 primary teeth that usually have all
grown in by the age of three. Ten on the top and the same
number on the bottom.

Adult teeth often start growing in at about age six,
and keep coming in at different times.
Sometimes they push out a primary tooth and
other times they grow in funny and need help.
People usually end up with 32 adult teeth.

Permanent molar teeth grow in every six years, so at
around age 6, 12 and 18 another set of chewing teeth
can be expected. These are called the first, second and
third molars. The third molars are called wisdom teeth.

Habits like thumb sucking and mouth breathing can cause
problems with the teeth and a dentist should be asked
for advice.

Tooth decay is a disease where the hard part of the tooth becomes softened or 'rotten'. The hole is often called a cavity and if the dentist finds it soon enough it can often be fixed in a few minutes with a filling.

Bite problems often should be corrected early and regular checkups and orthodontic examinations are helpful.

Certain things can be harmful to your teeth such as sloppy brushing and flossing, drinking and eating too many things that contain sugar, and doing things that could lead to a nasty bump in the mouth.

Protective mouth guards for sports activities and full shields if applicable can greatly reduce the risk of tooth damage.

Fluoride is a medicine for the teeth that can reduce cavities, ask your hygienist for the latest recommendations that have the most benefits.

Ask your dental professional if you have any questions about your smile and remember don't wait until your tooth hurts before you visit your dentist!

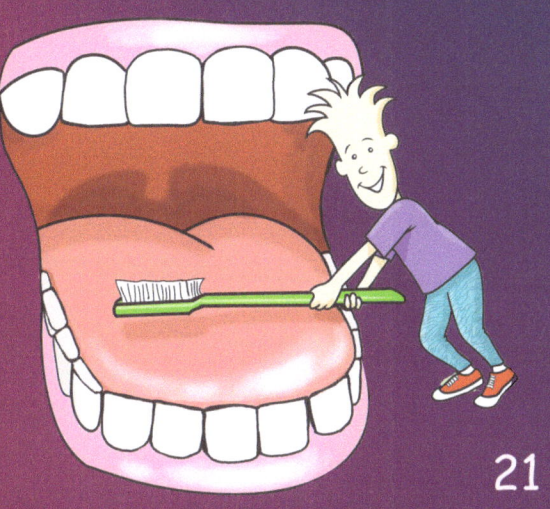

"DRAW YOUR OWN CARTOON VISIT TO THE DENTIST".

"DRAW YOUR OWN CARTOON VISIT TO THE DENTIST".

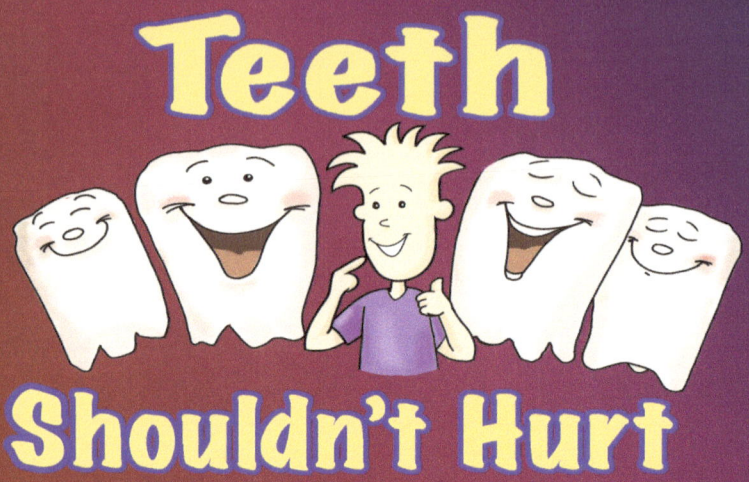

Teeth
Shouldn't Hurt

"I believe that one of the most important activities parents need to encourage and participate in with their child is the activity of reading. Results of a comprehensive study on reading completed by the National Commission on Reading strongly indicates that reading aloud to our children is the single most important intervention for developing their comprehension, literacy, and life skills. I would highly recommend this book as it can encourage your child to take their dental health seriously."

Tom Watson -Author- Man Shoes